Effective 5 Day Diets Guide + 57 Recipes

Military Diet, Blast Fat Detox Plan, Sirtfood, Super food Liver Detox, Paleo diet and others

Eric P. Garvin

Table of Contents

Introduction

If most people were honest, weight loss tends to stay at the top of our priorities list at any given time. Due to some reasons, many of us haven't achieved success yet by losing weight. It seems that you are reading this guide because you haven't achieved the desired results.

According to my experience as a diet and fitness specialist, I have made one important discovery that there is a thin line between success and failure when it comes to losing weight – TIME.

Most people want to lose weight quickly and to do it painlessly. Unfortunately, diets that guarantee fast weight loss are not only unsafe, but they only work over time when you keep a diet. In such a case it is better to keep The Military Diet. It isn't necessary to cut calories or starve to lose extra pounds. It's the conscious coupling of healthy food and chemical reaction with various processes in your body that helps to achieve incredible results.

The diet includes major food groups, which provide your body with the necessary nutrition. The best part is that you will have a chance to notice results during the first day of keeping this diet.

In addition to the Military Diet, we are also going to explore other diets that are related to it. These diets can help you to lose excess pounds once and for all. There was testing of numerous detox and low-calorie diets on the market.

The best thing about these diets is that they are based on *fresh and natural food*. It means that your body will never have a lack of necessary nutrients.

The six diets include:

The Three-Day Blast Fat Detox Plan – This diet is the perfect chance to give your body a quick wake-up call and to help by getting rid of excess toxins that can hamper the functioning of your vital organs. Over these three days, you are going to not only notice extra energy, but to revitalize health as well.

The Three-Day Sirtfood Diet – This diet is based on the usage of special proteins, which are also called sirtuins. The main aim of this diet is to help you to boost metabolism and build a fat-burning furnace in your body.

The Super food Liver Detox Diet Program – So many people fight against their overweight, not knowing what actually the cause of overweight is. If you have tried all diets in the book, eaten right and exercised regularly and still don't have results of your hard work, then most likely, your liver is the culprit. This diet will help cleanse your liver and bring it back to the great shape and you will lose weight.

The Negative Calorie Diet – Just as the name suggests, this diet focuses on negative-calorie food that will create a caloric deficiency in your body and help you to shed the pounds.

The Paleo Diet – This diet takes us back to eating real and not processed food that our ancestors had eaten. It uses 100% natural food to nourish your body and this makes it possible to lose sustainable weight.

The Whole Foods Diet – This diet is very similar to the Paleo Diet as it lays emphasis on eating food exactly, how it is conceived by nature. However, it also prohibits eating of a certain food to lose weight significantly.

Now, when we have an idea of what to expect, let's do it!

Military Diet

How The Military Diet works

By contrast with many diets that you have probably tried without any significant results, the Military Diet works actually. The reason is not simply, because it has been created by some of the best US Military nutritionists to get their soldiers in their best shape, it's because, if you keep the diet, you will get results.

There are three fundamental reasons why this diet works:

It is a low-calorie diet

A typical woman expends 1800 calories every day before engaging in any form of exercises. By keeping The Military Diet, you consume only 1000 calories during a day. This means that you automatically activate a calorie deficit mode.

A pound of fat is equal to 3500 calories, and you should burn 3500 calories to lose a pound. This diet works, because you consume fewer calories than you burn for three days in a week.

It is a special type of intermittent fasting

The fact that the Military Diet dictates 1000 or fewer calories in a day makes it a form of fasting, and fasting changes the dynamics of the body. For instance, it lowers the levels of produced insulin, which is a good thing, because it reduces the risk of diabetes aside from weight loss and a higher metabolic rate.

Fasting transitions help you to activate recovery mode rather than growth mode. Therefore, it utilizes much of your stored fat.

Intermittent fasting is a great and healthy way of inducing weight loss.

All food in The Military Diet boosts the fat-burning process

Grapefruit helps to start your liver into an active fat-burning mode, while high-protein foods like tuna require to produce more energy for their digestion. Each of the foods in the Military Diet will help your body to use more energy and to lose weight quickly.

Three-Day Military Diet

Day 1

Breakfast:

- 1 slice whole-wheat toast with 2 tablespoons of natural peanut butter
- ½ grapefruit
- 1 cup (250ml) of caffeinated tea or coffee

Lunch:

- 1/2 cup of tuna
- 1 slice of whole-wheat toast
- 1 cup of caffeinated tea or coffee

Dinner:

- 3 ounces of meat at choice
- 1 cup of green beans
- 1 apple
- 1/2 banana
- 1 cup of vanilla ice cream

Day 2

Breakfast:

- 1 slice of whole-wheat toast
- 1 egg (any style)
- 1/2 banana

Lunch:

- 1 hard-boiled egg
- 1 cup of cottage cheese
- 5 saltine crackers

Dinner:

- 2 hot dogs (without buns)
- 1/2 banana
- 1/2 cup of carrots
- 1 cup of broccoli
- 1/2 cup of vanilla ice cream

Day 3

Breakfast:

- 1 small apple
- 1 slice of cheddar cheese
- 5 saltine crackers

Lunch:

- 1 slice of whole-wheat toast
- 1 hard-boiled egg

Dinner:

- 1/2 banana
- 1 cup of tuna
- 1/2 cup of vanilla ice cream

Three-Day Blast Fat Detox Diet

Our Three Day Blast Fat Detox Plan is the perfect way to restore your health. It involves natural and whole foods that are high in fibre, which will not only keep you full until your next meal, but will also help to eliminate waste from your body, leaving you feeling energized and fresh.

During this three-day flat belly program, you'll:

- Drink a warm glass of Wake up Flat Belly Drink within the first 30 minutes of waking up;
- Drink at least 4 litres of water during the day;
- Drink a glass of iced green tea before going to bed.

You'll need every day:

- 1 flat belly, fresh juice
- 2-3 flat belly smoothies
- 2 flat belly soups

4 litres (16 cups) of water

NOTE: If you feel like you need "real food" instead of soups and smoothies for three days, eat something light for dinner such as an egg-white.

3-Day Blast Fat Detox Plan

Day 1

Breakfast: 1 Serving Super Cleansing Smoothie

Lunch: 1 Serving Fat Burner Veggie Soup

Dinner: 1 Serving Red Onion & Apple Soup

Day 2

Breakfast: 1 Serving Super Cleansing Smoothie

Lunch: 1 Serving Fat Burner Veggie Soup

Dinner: 1 Serving Red Onion & Apple Soup

Day 3

Breakfast: 1 Serving Kale Spinach Berry Smoothie

Lunch: 1 Serving Hot & Sour Flat-Belly Soup

Dinner: 1 Serving Broccoli Detox Soup

The Blast Belly Fat Breakfast Recipes

Super Cleansing Smoothie

Yields: 1 Serving

Total Time: 5 Minutes

Preparation Time: 5 Minutes

Cook Time: N/A

Ingredients

- 1 tablespoon of ground chia seeds or flax seeds
- 1 cup of baby kale
- 4 tablespoons of fresh lemon juice
- 1 organic apple, unpeeled, cored
- 1/3 cup of chopped parsley
- 1 stalk celery
- 1/4 teaspoon of ground cinnamon
- 1 1/4 cups of chilled water
- Ice cubes

Directions

Combine all ingredients in a blender and blend until a very smooth paste is obtained. Enjoy!

Kale Spinach Berry Smoothie

Yield: 1 Serving

Ingredients

- 1 cup of baby spinach
- 1 cup of chopped kale
- 1 cup of frozen blueberries
- 1/2 banana, peeled and cut into chunks
- 1 apple, cored and quartered
- 2 cups of water
- 1-2 packets with stevia

Directions

Combine together all the ingredients in a blender and blend until a very smooth paste is obtained. Enjoy!

Apple Dandelion Green Smoothie

Yield: 1 Serving

Ingredients

- 2 cups of dandelion greens
- 1/2 cup of frozen cranberries
- 1/2 banana, peeled
- 1 apple, cored
- 1 pear, cored
- 8 ounces of filtered water

Directions

Combine all ingredients in a blender until a creamy and smooth paste is obtained. Serve right away!

The Blast Belly Fat Lunch & Dinner Recipes

Fat Burner Veggie Soup

Yield: 8 Servings

Ingredients

- 4 cups of navy beans
- 1 sweet potato, peeled, diced
- 1 clove garlic, minced
- 1 small yellow onion, diced
- 1 stalk celery, diced
- 3 carrots, peeled and sliced
- 1 teaspoon of paprika
- 1/8 teaspoon of allspice
- 1/2 teaspoon of black pepper
- ¼ teaspoon of sea salt
- 2 cups of diced tomatoes
- 4 cups of vegetable broth
- 1 bay leaf
- 4 cups of baby spinach
- 1 teaspoon of extra-virgin olive oil

Directions

Combine all ingredients, except olive oil and spinach, in a slow cooker. Cook, covered, for about 7 hours or until the veggies are tender; remove the pot from heat and mash the ingredients with a fork. Return the pot and continue cooking for 1 hour more. Stir in spinach and cook for about 5 minutes or until it is wilted. Serve drizzled with a splash of extra virgin olive oil. Enjoy!

Hot & Sour Flat-Belly Soup

Yield: 4 Servings

Ingredients

- 2 tablespoons of extra-virgin olive oil
- 1 red onion, sliced
- 2 jalapeño peppers, seeds removed and diced
- 4 cups of sliced green cabbage
- 1 carrot, peeled and chopped
- 4 cups of crushed tomatoes
- 2 cups of chicken breast, shredded
- 4 cups of vegetable broth
- 3 tablespoons of apple cider vinegar
- 2 tablespoons of brown sugar
- ½ teaspoon of salt
- ¼ teaspoon of black pepper

Directions

Heat extra virgin olive oil in a skillet, which is set over medium heat;   stir red onion, jalapenos, cabbage and carrot; sauté for about 7 minutes or until it is almost tender.

Stir in tomatoes, chicken breast, broth, apple cider vinegar, brown sugar, salt and pepper until they are well-combined. Simmer, stirring frequently, for about 20 minutes. Serve hot.

Red Onion & Apple Soup

Yield: 6 Servings

Ingredients

- 1 tablespoon of canola oil
- 1 cup of chopped red onion
- 3 organic apples, diced
- 6 cups of vegetable broth
- 1/2 tablespoon of chopped fresh rosemary
- 1 leek, chopped
- 1/2 tablespoon of fresh thyme
- A pinch of cayenne pepper
- A pinch of sea salt

Directions

In a medium saucepan heat canola oil; stir in onion and sauté for about 4 minutes or until it is fragrant and golden.

Stir in broth and bring the mixture to a gentle boil.

Stir in the apples and simmer for about 10 minutes. Stir in rosemary, leek, thyme, cayenne pepper and salt. Serve right away.

Cleansing Detox Soup

Yield: 4 Servings

Total Time: 35 Minutes

Preparation Time: 15 Minutes

Cook Time: 20 Minutes

Ingredients

- 1/4 cup of water
- 2 cloves garlic, minced
- 1/2 of a red onion, diced
- 1 tablespoon of fresh ginger, peeled and minced
- 1 cup of chopped tomatoes
- 1 small head of broccoli, florets
- 3 medium carrots, diced
- 3 celery stalks, diced
- 6 cups of water
- 1/4 teaspoon of cinnamon
- 1 teaspoon of turmeric
- 1/8 teaspoon of cayenne pepper
- Sea salt
- Freshly ground black pepper
- Juice of 1 lemon

- 1 cup of purple cabbage, chopped
- 2 cups of kale, torn in pieces

Directions

Bring a large pot of water to a gentle boil over medium heat. Add garlic and onion and cook for about 2 minutes, stirring periodically. Stir in fresh ginger, tomatoes, broccoli, carrots, celery and continue cooking for 3 minutes more. Stir in cinnamon, turmeric, cayenne pepper, sea salt and black pepper.

Add in ½ cup water and bring the mixture to a rolling boil; reduce heat and simmer for about 15 minutes or until the veggies are tender. Stir in lemon juice, cabbage, and kale during the last 2 minutes of cooking. Serve hot or warm.

Broccoli Detox Soup

Yield: 2 Servings

Total Time: 20 Minutes

Preparation Time: 5 Minutes

Cook Time: 15 Minutes

Ingredients

- 1 teaspoon of coconut oil
- 2 garlic cloves, crushed
- 1 onion, diced
- 2 cups of broccoli florets
- 1 carrot, chopped
- 1 parsnip, chopped
- 2 celery stalks, diced
- 2 cups of filtered water
- 1 cup of greens (beet greens, spinach, kale or any other available)
- Juice of ½ lemon
- 1 tablespoon of chia seeds
- ½ teaspoon of sea salt
- 1 teaspoon of coconut milk, for serving
- Toasted mixed seeds and nuts, for serving

Directions

Heat coconut oil in a soup pot, which is set over low heat; stir in garlic, onion, broccoli, celery sticks, parsnip and carrot; cook for about 5 minutes, stirring frequently.

Stir in water and bring the mixture to a gentle boil; cover and simmer for about 7 minutes or until veggies are tender.

Stir in the greens and transfer to a food processor or blender; add lemon juice, chia seeds, sea salt and pulse until a very smooth paste is obtained.

Stir in coconut milk and sprinkle with toasted seeds and serve right away.

Three-Day Sirt Food Weight Loss Diet Plan

Introduction

Simply put, the sirtfood diet bases on eating foods, which are rich in nutrients. The nutrients interact with a special group of proteins that are called sirtuin, which is found in our bodies. Commonly numbered SIRT1 to SIRT7, sirtuins help the body to burn fat, boost metabolism, regulate internal bacteria and provide longer life of mammals.

The top 20 Sirtfoods

Many foods contain nutrients that activate sirtuin, but some contain a higher content of activators than others.

The top twenty sirtfoods include:

- Buckwheat
- Chilies
- Extra virgin olive oil
- Capers
- Medjool dates

- Citrus fruit
- Cocoa
- Coffee
- Celery
- Kale
- Rocket
- Green tea
- Red wine
- Red onion
- Lovage
- Red chicory
- Turmeric
- Soy
- Strawberries
- Walnuts

So How Does The Sirtfood Diet Work?

The Sirtfood Diet is a calorie-based diet. Many people are attracted to the diet, because it allows for consuming delicious and sinful foods, such as chocolate and red wine.

Health Benefits of Sirtfood Diet Program

Think of the Sirtfood Diet like of pushing the 'reset' button with your overall health, relationship with food and your lifestyle habits.

The most important food condition is actually quite simple: the food, which you eat, will either impact positively or negatively on your health. There's no grey area, it's either black or white – every bite you take is either nourishing your body or harming it, making you fat and sick.

This makes everything so simple, right? You only eat the foods that are going to impact positively on your life.

The Sirtfood Diet will turn you into an experimental guinea pig, so you can do some introspective work and figure yourself out.

The Three-Day SirtFood Diet Plan

Day 1

Breakfast: 1 Serving Sirty Breakfast Muesli

AM Snack: 1 cup (250ml) Citrus, Blueberry & Rosemary Mocktail

Lunch: 1 Serving Red Onion and Kale Dhal w/ Buckwheat

PM Snack: 1 cup (250ml)Citric Blueberry Slush

Dinner: 1 Serving Salmon with celery Salad, Rocket and Caramelized Chicory

Day 2

Breakfast: 1 Serving Sirty Breakfast Muesli

AM Snack: 1 cup (250ml) Citrus, Blueberry & Rosemary Mocktail

Lunch: 1 Serving Red Onion and Kale Dhal w/ Buckwheat

PM Snack: 1 cup (250ml) Citrus, Blueberry & Rosemary Mocktail

Dinner: 1 Serving Beef with Roasted Potatoes, Red Onions, & red wine

Day 3

Breakfast: 1 Serving Oat-Black-currant Yogurt Swirl

AM Snack: 1 cup (250ml) Citric Blueberry Slush

Lunch: 1 Serving Green Salad with Red Onion, Orange & Avocado

PM Snack: 1 cup Red Wine, Hot Chocolate

Dinner: 1 Serving Chicken w/Red Onions & Kale (Served with Chili-Tomato Salsa)

Sirt food Breakfast Recipes

Sirty Breakfast Muesli

Yield: 4 Servings

Total Time: 10 Minutes

Preparation Time: 10 Minutes

Cook Time: N/A

Ingredients:

- 2 cups of plain Greek yoghurt
- 2 cups of hulled and chopped strawberries
- ¼ cup of cocoa nibs
- ½ cup of chopped walnut
- 1 cup of pitted and chopped Medjool dates
- ¼ cup of coconut flakes
- ¼ cup of buckwheat puffs
- ½ cup of buckwheat flakes

Directions

In a large bowl, mix all the ingredients, except strawberries and yoghurt; let stand for at least

10 minutes. Stir in yoghurt and strawberries and serve.

Healthy Sirtfood Pancake

Yield: 6-8 Pancakes

Total Time: 45 Minutes

Preparation Time: 25 Minutes

Cook Time: 20 Minutes

For the pancakes you will need:

- 1 cup of milk
- ½ cup of buckwheat flour
- 1 large egg
- 1 tbsp. extra virgin olive oil

For the chocolate sauce

- 1 tbsp. extra virgin olive oil
- 1 tbsp. double cream
- ½ cup of milk
- ½ cup of chopped dark chocolate

To serve

- ½ cup of chopped walnuts
- 1 ½ cups of chopped strawberries

Directions

Make pancake batter: mix all ingredients, except extra virgin olive oil, in a blender and blend until a very smooth paste is obtained.

Make chocolate sauce: in a heatproof bowl, melt chocolate over a pan of simmering water; when it will melt, whisk in milk, double cream and extra virgin olive oil; keep warm.

Make the pancakes: place a heavy frying pan over medium heat; heat olive oil and add the pancake batter in the centre and spread to cover the entire surface. Cook the pancakes for about 1 minute per side or until they brown on the edges.

Transfer the cooked pancakes to a plate and keep warm.

To serve, spoon a good amount of the sauce over the pancakes and sprinkle with chopped walnuts. Enjoy!

Oat-Black-currant Yogurt Swirl

Yield: 2 Servings

Total Time: 25 Minutes

Preparation Time: 15 Minutes

Cook Time: 5 Minutes

Ingredients

- ¼ cup of oats
- 1 cup of natural yoghurt
- ½ cup of black currants
- 2 tbsp. caster sugar
- ½ cup of water

Directions

Mix water, black-currant and castor sugar in a pan and bring to a gentle boil. Reduce the heat to a simmer and cook for about 5 minutes; turn off the heat and let cool. Refrigerate the black-currant compote until it is ready to use.

In a large bowl, mix the oats and yoghurt.

To serve, divide the black-currant compote between two bowls and top each with oat mixture; with a cocktail stick, swirl the black-currant compote through the oat-yoghurt mixture and serve immediately.

SirtFood Diet Lunch Recipes

Green Salad with Red Onion, Orange & Avocado

Yield: 6 Servings

Total Time: 15 Minutes

Preparation Time: 15 Minutes

Cook Time: N/A

Ingredients

- 2 medium avocados, sliced
- 2 medium navel oranges, segmented and segments squeezed into juice
- 1/2 medium red onion, thinly sliced
- 1/4 cup of extra-virgin olive oil
- 1 small clove garlic, finely chopped
- 1 tsp. Dijon mustard
- 2 tbsp. sherry vinegar
- 1/8 tsp. salt
- 1 head Romaine lettuce, chopped

Directions

In a bowl, combine garlic, vinegar, 1 tablespoon of orange juice, mustard and salt; whisk in extra virgin olive oil until a smooth and emulsified paste is obtained.

In a salad bowl, combine avocado, red onion, lettuce and strained orange segments; drizzle with the dressing and toss until it is well-combined. Serve right away.

Red Wine-Mushroom Stew w/ Kale

Yield: 4 Servings

Total Time: 1 Hour 10 Minutes

Preparation Time: 20 Minutes

Cook Time: 50 Minutes

Ingredients

- 1 cup of uncooked wild rice
- 1 cup of sliced red onion
- 6 oz. Portobello mushrooms, sliced
- ½ cup of red wine
- ½ cup of miso paste
- 4 cups of vegetable broth
- 10 oz. kale, chopped
- 3 cups of water
- 2 cups of sliced carrots
- ½ tsp. red pepper chilli flakes
- 2 tbsp. garlic powder
- 2 tbsp. ground cumin
- 1 tsp. black pepper

Directions

Blend together 1 cup of water and miso paste in a blender until a smooth paste is obtained; transfer it to a soup pot. Stir in the chilli flakes, garlic powder, cumin, rice, broth and the remaining water; bring the mixture to a gentle boil. Reduce heat and simmer for about 30 minutes or until rice is tender.

Stir in kale cook for about 4 minutes or until kale is wilted. Remove from heat and season with salt. Serve right away.

Red Onion and Kale Dhal w/ Buckwheat

Yield: 1 Serving

Total Time: 1 Hour 5 Minutes

Preparation Time: 15 Minutes

Cook Time: 50 Minutes

Ingredients

- 1 tsp. extra virgin olive oil
- 1 chilli, finely chopped
- 40g red onion, finely chopped
- 1 tsp. finely chopped fresh ginger
- 1 garlic clove, finely chopped
- 1 tsp. mustard seeds
- 2 tsp. ground turmeric
- 1 tsp. mild curry powder
- ¼ cup of chopped kale
- ¼ cup of coconut milk
- ¼ cup of red lentils, rinsed
- 1 ¼ cup of vegetable stock
- ¼ cup of buckwheat

Directions

Heat extra virgin olive oil in a frying pan, which is set over medium heat; add mustard seeds and fry until the seeds start popping; stir in red onion, chilli, garlic and ginger and cook for about 10 minutes or until tender condition. Stir 1 teaspoon turmeric and curry powder and continue cooking for about 3 minutes. Add stock and bring the mixture to a gentle boil.

Add lentils and reduce heat to a simmer; simmer for about 30 minutes or until lentils are tender. Stir in coconut milk and kale and continue cooking for about 5 minutes or until kale is wilted.

Meanwhile, follow packet instructions to cook buckwheat; drain and serve with dhal.

Sirt food Diet Dinner Recipes

Salmon with celery Salad, Rocket and Caramelized Chicory

Yield: 1 Serving

Total Time: 25 Minutes

Preparation Time: 15 Minutes

Cook Time: 10 Minutes

Ingredients

- 150g skinless salmon fillet
- 1 tbsp. extra virgin olive oil
- 20g red onion, thinly sliced
- 1 tbsp. capers
- Juice of ¼ lemon
- 10g parsley
- 5g celery leaves
- 50g rocket
- 100g cherry tomatoes, halved
- ¼ avocado, peeled, stoned and diced
- 1 head (70g) chicory, halved lengthways
- 2 tsp. brown sugar

Directions

Preheat your oven to 450°F.

Make the dressing: combine capers, lemon juice, parsley and 2 teaspoons of extra virgin olive oil in a food processor; process until a smooth condition.

Make the salad: combine avocado, red onion, celery, tomatoes and rocket in a salad bowl; set aside.

Rub fish with oil and sear in a hot frying pan for about 1 minute until caramelized condition; transfer to a baking tray and roast in the oven for about 6 minutes.

In a small bowl, mix the remaining oil with brown sugar and brush over the cut sides of chicory; arrange chicory, cut side down and cook on a hot frying pan for about 3 minutes or until caramelized and tender condition.

To serve, toss the lemon dressing in the salad and serve with caramelized chicory and salmon.

Chicken w/Red Onions & Kale (Served with Chili-Tomato Salsa)

Yield: 1 Serving

Total Time: 40 Minutes

Preparation Time: 20 Minutes

Cook Time: 20 Minutes

Ingredients:

- 120g chicken breast, skinless, boneless
- 1 large red onion, sliced
- 1 tbsp. extra virgin olive oil
- 2 tsp. ground turmeric
- 1 tsp. chopped ginger
- 50g kale, chopped
- Juice of 1⁄4 lemon
- 50g buckwheat

For the salsa

- 1 large tomato, finely chopped
- ½ cup parsley, finely chopped
- 1 tbsp. capers, finely chopped
- 1 bird's eye chili, finely chopped
- Juice of 1⁄4 lemon

Directions

Make the salsa: mix chopped tomato, capers, chilli, lemon juice and parsley in a large bowl.

Preheat your oven to 450°F.

In a large bowl, mix lemon juice, 1 teaspoon turmeric and a splash of extra virgin olive oil; add the chicken and stir to combine well. Marinate for about 10 minutes.

Set an ovenproof pan over medium heat and add the chicken; cook for about 4 minutes per side or until it is lightly browned. Transfer to the preheated oven and bake for about 10 minutes, remove from the oven and keep warm.

In the meantime, steam kale in a steamer for about 5 minutes.

Fry ginger and red onion in a splash of extra virgin olive oil until tender condition; stir in kale and cook for about 1 minute.

Follow package instructions to cook buckwheat with the remaining turmeric.

Serve the buckwheat with chicken, veggies and salsa.

Beef with Roasted Potatoes, Red Onions, & red wine

Yield: 1 Serving

Total Time: 1 Hour 55 Minutes

Preparation Time: 15 Minutes

Cook Time: 1 Hour 40 Minutes

Ingredients

- 150g beef steak
- 1 tbsp. extra virgin olive oil
- ¼ cup of red wine
- 100g potatoes, peeled and cut into
- ¼ cup of sliced red onion
- 1 garlic clove, finely chopped
- 50g kale, sliced
- 1 tbsp. parsley, finely chopped
- 1 tsp. tomato purée
- ½ cup beef stock
- 1 tsp. corn flour
- 1 tbsp. water

Directions

Preheat your oven to 450°F.

Boil potatoes in water for about 5 minutes; drain and transfer to a roasting tin. Drizzle with a teaspoon of extra virgin olive oil and roast in the oven for about 45 minutes, turning every 10 minutes. Remove from oven and mix with chopped parsley.

Heat a teaspoon of extra virgin olive oil in a pan over medium heat and sauté red onion for about 7 minutes or until caramelized condition.

In a steamer, steam kale for about 3 minutes.

Sauté garlic in ½ teaspoon of oil for about 1 minute or until tender condition; add kale and cook for about 32 minutes.

Coat beef with the remaining oil and fry it in a pan over medium heat; remove from heat and set aside.

Add red wine to the pan and cook until it is reduced by half and is syrupy. Stir in the tomato puree and stock and bring the mixture to a gentle boil; make the cornflour paste by dissolving cornflour into a tablespoon of water. Stir the cornflour paste into the mixture and cook until the sauce is thick.

Serve beef with the red wine sauce, onion rings, kale and roasted potatoes.

SirtFood Juices and Drinks

Sirty Juice

Yield: 1 Serving

Total Time: 5 Minutes

Preparation Time: 5 Minutes

Cook Time: N/A

Ingredients

- ½ tsp. Matcha powder
- ½ lemon, juiced
- ½ green apple, juiced
- 3 green celery stalks, juiced
- 1 cup of rocket/arugula, juiced
- 2 cups of kale, juiced
- 1 tbsp. parsley, juiced

Directions

Combine the juices together in a glass and stir in matcha powder until it is well-combined. Serve right away!

Red Wine, Hot Chocolate

Yield: 4 Servings

Total Time: 10 Minutes

Preparation Time: 5 Minutes

Cook Time: 5 Minutes

Ingredients

- ⅔ cup of dry red wine
- ⅔ cup of semi-sweet chocolate chips
- 2 tbsp. sugar
- ½ cup of milk
- ½ tsp. vanilla extract
- 1/8 tsp. salt

Directions

In a small saucepan, which is set over medium-low heat, combine wine, chocolate chips, milk and sugar; heat, stirring, for about 5 minutes or until chocolate is completely melted.

Remove from heat and stir in salt and vanilla; pour into serving mugs and enjoy!

Citric Blueberry Slush

Yield: 6 Servings

Total Time: 5 Minutes

Preparation Time: 5 Minutes

Cook Time: N/A

Ingredients

- 1-1/2 cups of frozen blueberries
- 1-1/2 cups of fresh orange juice
- 2 tbsp. lime juice
- 2 tbsp. lemon juice
- 1/2 cup of raw honey
- 1 cup of crushed ice

Directions

In a blender, combine honey, lime, lemon and orange juices; blend it until honey is dissolved; add ice cubes, blueberries and puree. Pour into serving glasses and garnish with a lime or lemon wedge. Enjoy!

Citrus, Blueberry & Rosemary Mocktail

Yield: 1 Serving

Total Time: 1 Hour 20 Minutes

Preparation Time: 1 Hour 10 Minutes

Cook Time: 10 Minutes

Ingredients

For rosemary syrup:

- 4 springs fresh rosemary
- ¼ cup of water
- ½ cup of sugar

For cocktail:

- ½ ounce fresh lime juice
- 1.5 ounces of rosemary syrup
- crushed ice
- Lime slice & fresh blueberries

Directions

Make the syrup: combine water, sugar and rosemary in a pan; simmer for about 10 minutes or until sugar is completely dissolved. Cover the pan and steep for at least 1 hour.

Make the mocktail: Combine lime juice and rosemary syrup in a shaker and shake to mix well. Pour into serving glasses and stir in ice cubes. Garnish with fresh blueberries and lime slices.

Superfood Liver Detox Diet Program

The Liver Cleanse – The Weight Loss Secret You've Never Heard

If you can't shrink down your waistline, regardless of which healthy products you eat or how much you train, the problem may reside not in your waistline, but in another organ.

Most of us are guilty of not giving much thought to our livers, except maybe when thinking about the third shot of tequila, but its harmful effect is essential to your general health and weight. Your liver is perhaps the most worked organ in your body. It filters out toxins such as alcohol and medicines as well as byproducts of the digestive process such as ammonia. It plays a big role in regulating glucose, blood sugar, blood pressure, insulin, immunity, blood cholesterol and testosterone. The liver helps in digestion by generating bile, which helps to break down fat and absorb fat particles and water-soluble minerals and vitamins.

Because of this extensive to-do list, your liver needs some care. When it gets overworked, toxic compounds start building up, which cause inflammation and is the main culprit of weight gain and obesity.

Why Should You Cleanse Your Liver?

Many people disregard liver cleansing, saying that the human body is self-sustaining. While this is true, we cannot assume the fact that every day we see people suffering from obesity, heart diseases and other chronic illnesses. These illnesses are mostly caused by inflammation, which is your body's way of responding to foreign material that it's not able to eliminate. With the increased levels of toxic content in our environment, we have no choice, but to help our bodies eliminate the excessive fat accumulation.

By cleansing your liver, you are empowering it to deal with all kinds of toxins. Here are some of the benefits you gain from cleansing your liver regularly.

Sustainable Weight Loss

Bile is essential to the breakdown of fats in your body. Cleansing your liver encourages bile production, thus optimizing the fat-breakdown process. You want to cleanse your liver as your first step in trying to lose weight.

Increased Energy

Some by-products, which are produced by the liver, are nutrients that your body uses. However, when you have too much toxic content or liver stones, these prevent some nutrients from entering into the bloodstream. When this happens, you start to feel tired and slack. Cleansing your liver helps nutrients to enter and leave your liver without being blocked by toxins. That's why you start to notice improved energy levels.

Boost Your Immune Function

As your liver mainly eliminates toxins from your body, improving its function of eliminating toxins will also improve your overall immunity. It doesn't have to keep fighting off toxins and it can now focus on protecting your body from diseases.

Supports Your Entire Body's Detoxification

Cleansing your liver doesn't just stop only at your liver, it cleanses your entire organism from toxin accumulation. Remember that it's your liver's job to eliminate toxins, meaning that the amount of toxins in your liver is usually fewer than in your whole body. Therefore, by cleansing your liver, you are enabling it to work better at eliminating the toxic accumulation in your body.

Increased Vitality

Removing toxins from your liver restores its maximum efficiency. With increased bile production and improved fat breakdown, you will find it easier to lose weight with the help of exercises and healthy eating and the new joy, which you are going to experience, will know no boundaries.

Other benefits of liver cleansing include healthy and younger-looking skin and hair, improved health and a better understanding of how your body works. The moment, when you notice that you take care of your liver and whole body in general, you feel so much better and will never go back to your old mentality of dieting.

Of all the basic principles of our lives, health is perhaps the most important. Start the liver cleansing diet today and reap the benefits of pure health!

General Healthy Liver Diet

- Drink a warm glass of water immediately after waking up and before going to bed.
- Drink at least 8 glasses of water during the day.
- No dairy, grains, sugar or alcohol.
- Avoid processed/packaged food, corn syrup, trans fats, hydrogenated fats, dried or canned fruits, juices and gluten.
- Eat at least one kind of product during each meal from the superfood list, which is mentioned above.

The 3-Day Liver Detox Meal Plan

Day 1

Breakfast: 1 Serving Superfood Detox Pancakes

AM Snack: Handful toasted almonds

Lunch: 1 Serving Avocado Grapefruit Edamame Salad

PM Snack: 1 pear

Dinner: 1 Serving Turkey & Quinoa Salad

Day 2

Breakfast: 1 Serving Superfood Detox Pancakes

AM Snack: Handful toasted almonds

Lunch: 1 Serving Avocado Grapefruit Edamame Salad

PM Snack: Handful blueberries

Dinner: 1 Serving Superfood Salmon Salad

Day 3

Breakfast: 1 Serving Beet Quinoa w/ Orange

AM Snack: 1 small apple

Lunch: 1 Serving Swiss Chard Wrap

PM Snack: 1 cup (250ml) fresh grapefruit juice

Dinner: 1 Serving Shrimp Salad w/ Grapefruit and Avocado

Superfood Detox Breakfast Recipes

Superfood Detox Pancakes

Yield: 1 Serving

Total Time: 15-17 Minutes

Preparation Time: 5 Minutes

Cook Time: 10-12 Minutes

Ingredients

- 1/3 cup of rolled oats
- 1/2 teaspoon of cinnamon
- 1/2 teaspoon of baking powder
- 2 tablespoons of ground flax
- 1/2 medium ripe banana
- 3 large egg-whites
- 2 cups of spinach
- 1/2 teaspoon of vanilla extract

Directions

Set a nonstick skillet over medium heat; coat with olive oil.

In a food processor or blender, blend the oats into fine flour; transfer to a bowl and stir in the remaining dry ingredients.

In a blender, combine banana, egg-whites, spinach and vanilla, blend until a very smooth paste is obtained.

Add the banana mixture into the dry ingredients and stir to form a batter.

Spoon batter onto the heated skillet, forming four pancakes. Cook for about 6 minutes per side or until it is browned.

Transfer the pancakes to a plate and top with fresh fruit and nuts.

Superfood Granola

Yield: 5 Cups (6 Servings)

Total Time: 3 Hours 20 Minutes + Soaking Time

Preparation Time: 20 Minutes

Cook Time: 3 Hours

Ingredients:

- 1 1/2 cups of soaked almonds and walnuts
- 1 cup of soaked sunflower seeds or a mix with pumpkin seeds
- 2 cups of soaked whole buckwheat (minimum 4hrs) preferably sprouted for 1-2 days
- 3 grated apples, (strain some of the juice from the grated apple)
- 1/2 cup of pureed dates, soaked for about 15 minutes
- 1/4 cup of dried prunes
- 1/2 cup of goji berries, soaked for nine minutes
- 1/2 cup of dry coconut flakes
- 1 teaspoon of vanilla

- 3 teaspoons of cinnamon
- 1/3 teaspoon of salt
- 1 tablespoon of cacao nibs
- 1 tablespoon of hulled hemp seeds

Instructions

Soak buckwheat for a minimum of 4 hours and rinse thoroughly.

Soak all the nuts and seeds for a minimum of 4 hours and rinse.

Soak dates in water enough to cover for a minimum of 15 minutes or until they are soft.

Soak the Goji berries in a sufficient amount of water to cover.

Chop or lightly put through your food processor the nuts and seeds. Maybe leave some whole nuts and seeds or until your desired consistency.

When all ingredients are soaked, rinse and add all together in a large bowl and mix well, use your hands for the easiest method.

Take the mixture and spread evenly over a baking tray and cook for 2-3 hours at

200°F/95°C or until it is dry. You may use a higher temperature for quicker cooking. To make this recipe raw, you may use a dehydrator at 105° F/55°C for 12-15 hours (turning over, when the top is totally dry).

After completely drying you can store it in an airtight container for a couple of weeks.

Serve with a nut or seed milk or eat as a dry snack.

Beet Quinoa w/ Orange

Yield: 2 Serving

Total Time: 35 Minutes

Preparation Time: 10 Minutes

Cook Time: 25 Minutes

Ingredients

- ½ red onion, thinly sliced
- 1 tablespoon of apple cider vinegar
- 2-3 beets
- 1 cup of quinoa
- 1 stalk celery, thinly sliced
- 1 teaspoon of grated ginger
- Extra virgin olive oil
- Juice of 1 lemon
- 1 small orange, thinly sliced
- ½ tsp. sea salt
- ½ tsp. freshly ground black pepper

Directions

Combine sliced onion and apple cider vinegar in a bowl; let soak for at least 10 minutes.

In the meantime, bring a pot of water to a gentle boil over medium heat. Rinse the beets and add to the boiling water; boil for about 10 minutes or until it is tenderly cooked, but not mushy.

Transfer the beets to a plate and reserve the cooking liquid; peel the cooked beets and chop thinly.

Follow package instructions to cook quinoa with using the reserved beet liquid. Season with salt during cooking. When it will be cooked, remove the quinoa from heat and set aside to cool.

In a large serving bowl, mix beets, quinoa, ginger and celery. Remove onion from the vinegar and stir into the bowl with the quinoa mixture.

Drizzle with extra virgin olive oil and lemon juice. Add orange slices and toss to mix well.

Season with salt and pepper for serving.

Superfood Detox Lunch Recipes

Swiss chard Wrap

Total Time: 20 Minutes

Yield: 4 Servings

Total Time: 20 Minutes

Preparation Time: 20 Minutes

Cook Time: 0 Minutes

Ingredients

- 4 large Swiss chard leaves
- 1 red bell pepper
- 1 avocado
- ¼ -1/3 cups of alfalfa sprouts
- 1 carrot
- 1 cucumber
- ½ lime
- 1/4 cup of pecans
- ½ tsp. minced garlic
- 1 tsp. cumin
- 1 tbsp. tamari

- ½ tsp. grated ginger
- 1 tsp. extra virgin olive oil
- Handful of alfalfa sprouts

Directions

To prepare Swiss chard, wash leaves, cut off the stiff white stem at the bottom and slice thinly to add to each wrap. Dry the leaves off with paper towels and using a knife, thinly slice down the central root (to make it easier to bend the leaves for wrapping).

Thinly slice all vegetables.

In a food processor, combine pecans, tamari, cumin, garlic, ginger and olive oil. Pulse until it is combined.

Place a collard leaf in front of you and layer nut mix, red pepper slices, avocado slices, cucumber, carrot and a drizzle of lime juice and alfalfa sprouts. Then wrap up the sides. I use a toothpick to keep the wrap together if it unwraps.

Avocado Grapefruit Edamame Salad

Yield: 3 Servings

Total Time: 15 Minutes

Preparation Time: 10 Minutes

Cook Time: N/A

For the Salad

- 1 small (or half of a large) ripe avocado, peeled and sliced
- 2 celery stalks, sliced
- 1 cup of shelled edamame
- 1 blood orange, segmented
- 1 grapefruit, segmented
- 2 cups of leafy greens

For the Dressing

- 1/4 cup plus 1 tablespoon of extra virgin olive oil
- 2 tablespoons of apple cider vinegar
- 1 tablespoon of gluten-free mustard
- 1 tablespoon of raw honey
- 3 tablespoons of diced shallots

- Sea salt and cracked black pepper, to taste

Directions

Combine all salad ingredients in a medium bowl.

Combine extra virgin olive oil, vinegar, mustard, raw honey, shallots, salt and pepper in a jar with a tight-fitting lid; seal and shake until it is well-blended.

Pour enough dressing over the salad and season with salt and pepper. Serve right away!

Green Super Detox Salad

Yield: 2 Servings

Total Time: 15 Minutes

Preparation Time: 15 Minutes

Cook Time: 0 Minutes

Ingredients

- 1 tbsp. extra virgin olive oil
- juice from 1 lemon
- 1/2 avocado
- 2 large cucumbers
- 1/4 cabbage
- 1/4 cup of chopped celery
- 1/8 cup of pistachios
- 1/4 head broccoli
- Sea salt and pepper

Directions

In a large bowl, combine extra virgin olive oil, lemon juice and avocado; mash with a fork until a smooth paste is obtained; season with salt and pepper and set aside.

Using a spiralizer or a veggie peeler, make the cucumber noodles.

Chop the remaining ingredients and toss them in a bowl with the cucumber noodles; add the avocado dressing and toss to combine well. Enjoy!

Superfood Detox Dinner Recipes

Shrimp Salad w/ Grapefruit and Avocado

Yield: 2 Servings

Total Time: 20 Minutes

Preparation Time: 10 Minutes

Cook Time: 10 Minutes

Ingredients

- 2 tablespoons of chilli oil
- 1 cup of shrimp
- ½ teaspoon of salt
- ½ teaspoon of pepper
- 1 avocado, cubed
- 1 grapefruit, cubed
- ¼ cup of lemon juice

Directions

Heat chilli oil in a saucepan, which is set over medium heat; add shrimp and cook until opaque and lightly browned condition.

Remove the pan from heat and season shrimp with sea salt and pepper.

In a serving bowl, pack avocado slices as tightly as possible, and then top with a layer of shrimp, grapefruit and drizzle with lemon juice. Serve, when shrimp is still hot!

Turkey & Quinoa Salad

Yield: 4 Servings

Total Time: 50 Minutes

Preparation Time: 20 Minutes

Cook Time: 30 Minutes

Ingredients

- 3 tablespoons of extra-virgin olive oil
- 1 1/2 cups of quinoa, rinsed
- Kosher salt
- 1 pound of turkey cutlets
- 3 tablespoons of chopped fresh tarragon and/or parsley
- Freshly ground pepper
- 1/2 small red onion, halved and sliced
- 1 1/2 pounds of assorted heirloom tomatoes, chopped
- 1 Chile pepper, seeded and chopped
- 4 Persian cucumbers, chopped
- 2 tablespoons of sherry vinegar

Directions

In a large skillet, which is set over medium-high heat, heat ½ tablespoon of extra virgin olive oil; stir in quinoa and cook, stirring continuously for about 4 minutes or until it is lightly toasted. Stir in salt and 4 cups of water; bring to a gentle boil, lower heat and simmer for about 15 minutes.

In a mixing bowl, toss together turkey, half of the herbs, a pinch of sea salt and pepper; set aside.

In a bowl, soak the sliced onion in cold water for at least 10 minutes.

In a separate bowl, toss together cucumbers, Chile, tomatoes, the remaining herbs, 1 ½ tablespoon of extra virgin olive oil, vinegar, sea salt and black pepper.

Drain the onion and stir into the tomato mixture.

Heat the remaining oil in a nonstick skillet, which is set over medium-high heat. Add turkey in batches and cook for about 3 minutes per side or until it is golden; drain on paper towels. Cut the cooked turkey into bite-sized pieces.

With a fork, fluff the cooked quinoa and divide among serving bowls; top each with turkey and tomato mixture.

Superfood Salmon Salad

Yield: 2 Servings

Total Time: 15 Minutes

Preparation Time: 5 Minutes

Cook Time: 10 Minutes

Ingredients

- 7 ounces of wild caught salmon fillets, skinned
- 7 ounces of broccoli
- 1 tablespoon of extra virgin olive oil
- 2 spring onions, thinly sliced
- ½ red chili, deseeded, chopped
- 1 tablespoon of mixed seeds (sesame seeds, sunflower seeds, pumpkin seeds, and linseeds)
- 1/8 cup of chopped nuts (almonds or brazil nuts)
- Juice of 1 orange
- 1 orange, zested

Directions

In a skillet, bring water to a gentle boil. Add fish and broccoli and cook 3 minutes or until fish is cooked and broccoli is tender.

Remove from heat and let cool a bit; drain the broccoli and set aside.

Heat extra virgin olive oil in a pan; add onions, chilli, seeds and nuts and fry for about 4 minutes or until it is golden.

Stir in orange juice and zest and season with sea salt and cracked black pepper.

Flake the fish into small pieces and mix with broccoli. Serve topped with nut and chilli mixture.

Flake the salmon into pieces, mix with the broccoli and sprinkle the chilli and nut mixture over the top.

The Negative Calorie Diet

What is the negative calorie diet?

The Negative Calorie Diet is an eating plan that is built on a 3-day plan and is aimed at jumpstarting healthy lifestyle changes over the long term. It starts with cleansing your body of all the toxins to feel the benefits of a nutrient-dense, organic and whole foods diet.

This is followed by delicious recipes that are built on protein and supplemented by organic negative calorie foods, superfoods and spices bursting with flavour, fat-burning and health-promoting results.

Negative calorie foods will help shed extra fat, boost your metabolism (the rate at which your body burns calories), and they will help you to stay fuller longer– meaning you're going to eat less food.

With the "Negative Calorie Diet, " we can finally say that we have solved the mystery of weight loss!

The Negative Calorie Diet Plan

Day 1

Breakfast: 1 Serving Berry Breakfast Bowl

AM Snack: 1 cup (250ml) fresh orange juice

Lunch: 1 Serving A Veggie Extravaganza!

PM Snack: 1 cup (250 ml) fresh grapefruit juice

Dinner: 1 Serving Citrusy Baked Salmon with Bulgur & Asparagus

Day 2

Breakfast: 1 Serving Berry Breakfast Bowl

AM Snack: 1 cup (250ml) fresh orange juice

Lunch: 1 Serving A Veggie Extravaganza!

PM Snack: 1 pear

Dinner: 1 Serving Herbed Chicken & Veggie Stir-Fry

Day 3

Breakfast: 1 Serving Healthy Herbed Frittata

AM Snack: Handful blueberries

Lunch: 1 Serving Minty Cucumber Salad

PM Snack: Handful toasted almonds

Dinner: 1 Serving Braised Chicken with Spring Veggies

Negative Calorie Breakfast Recipes

Berry Breakfast Bowl

Yields: 4 Servings

Total Time: 10 Minutes

Preparation Time: 10 Minutes

Cook Time: N/A

Ingredients

- ½ cup of strawberries
- ½ cup of blackberries
- ½ cup of raspberries
- ½ cup of blueberries
- 1/8 -1/4 cup of cooked quinoa
- 10 whole toasted almonds, roughly chopped
- 1 ½ tbsp. hemp hearts

Directions

Combine all the ingredients in a large bowl and toss well until it is evenly combined.

Divide the mixture into two bowls and top with a dollop of non-fat Greek yoghurt for a protein punch.

Yum!

Blueberry Quinoa Power Breakfast Muffins

Yields: 4 Servings

Total Time: 40 Minutes

Preparation Time: 20 Minutes

Cook Time: 20 Minutes

Ingredients

1 cup of oatmeal

1 cup of cooked quinoa, cooled

1/4 cup of raw brown sugar

¼ cup of natural honey

1/3 cup of flax seeds

1 tsp baking soda

1 tsp baking powder

2 tsp cinnamon

1 cup of fresh/frozen blueberries

1 tsp pure vanilla extract

½ cup of organic applesauce

¾ cup of non-fat plain Greek yoghurt

Directions

Start by setting your oven to 350°F and prepare a baking tin by lightly greasing it using non-stick cooking spray.

In a large bowl, combine all the dry ingredients until they are evenly combined then set aside. In a separate bowl, whisk together all the wet ingredients until you get an even consistency. Combine the dry ingredients well and pour in the wet ingredients.

Mix the ingredients until they are well-combined, but don't overwork the batter, else you will get the toughest muffins. Gently fold in the berries, then scoop the batter into the muffin tin, filling each cup about ¾ way full.

Bake for about 20 minutes or until an inserted toothpick emerges clean.

Remove from oven and cool on a wire rack. Serve warm.

Enjoy!

Healthy Herbed Frittata

Yields: 4 Servings

Total Time: 30 Minutes

Preparation Time: 20 Minutes

Cook Time: 10 Minutes

Ingredients

- 3 free range eggs, beaten
- 1 tsp extra virgin olive oil
- ¼ cup of water
- 1 cup of finely diced onion
- 2 tsp. freshly chopped mixed fresh herbs (dill, parsley, chervil and marjoram)
- 2 tbsp. low fat farmer's cheese
- Salt to taste
- Freshly ground black pepper to taste

Directions

Add the water to a small nonstick pan over medium-high heat and add in the diced onion. Bring to a boil and cook, covered, for 2 minutes. Uncover and continue cooking for about 2 minutes until all water evaporates.

Pour in the olive oil and cook the onions until they start browning for another 2 minutes or so.

Pour in the eggs and cook, stirring constantly and using a rubber spatula. Lift the edges so the uncooked egg flows underneath.

When the egg is almost set, lower the heat and sprinkle the pepper, herbs and salt. Top with the cheese and gently lift the eggs and add a tablespoon of water beneath it.

Cover and cook for 2 minutes and serve hot. Enjoy!

Negative Calorie Lunch Recipes

Minty Cucumber Salad

Yields: 4 Servings

Total Time: 20 Minutes + Chilling Time

Preparation Time: 20 Minutes

Cook Time: N/A

Ingredients

- 1 cucumber, very thinly sliced using a mandolin
- 2 carrots, thinly sliced
- ½ a Vidalia onion, thinly sliced
- 1/3 cup of white vinegar
- 3 packets of stevia (this is a zero calorie natural sweetener)
- Freshly squeezed juice of 1 lime
- 2 tbsp. fresh mint, chopped
- 1/3 cup of water
- Sea salt to taste
- Freshly ground pepper to taste

Directions

Sprinkle the sliced cucumbers with sea salt and let it stay for 20 minutes, then rinse out the salt and squeeze out the excess water.

Make the salad dressing and marinate the cucumber, carrots and onions and refrigerate for 2 hours.

Toss the salad ingredients with the chopped mint in a salad bowl.

Enjoy!

A Veggie Extravaganza!

Yields: 5 Servings

Total Time: 40 Minutes

Preparation Time: 15 Minutes

Cook Time: 25 Minutes

Ingredients

- 1 cup of celery, diced
- 2 cups of baby spinach
- 1 cup of cauliflower florets
- 2 cups of shredded cabbage
- 1 cup of green beans, cut into 1 inch pieces
- 2 cups of diced zucchini
- 1 onion, diced
- 1 cup of diced turnip
- 1 jalapeno, seeded and finely chopped
- 3 cloves garlic, finely grated
- Salt to taste
- Freshly ground pepper to taste
- 6 cups of low sodium vegetable stock – preferably home-made

Directions

Combine all the ingredients in a large saucepan or soup pot except for the baby spinach and place over medium to high heat.

Once it comes to a boil, reduce the heat to low and simmer for about 20 minutes, covered.

Adjust the seasonings, if they are desired, then stir in the baby spinach and cook or 30 seconds to one minute.

Serve in soup bowls.

Enjoy!

Berries & Greens Salad with Poppy Seed Dressing

Yields: 6 Servings

Total Time: 10 Minutes

Preparation Time: 10 Minutes

Cook Time: N/A

Ingredients

- 3 cups of arugula leaves, roughly torn
- 3 cups of watercress leaves
- 3 cups of strawberries, sliced
- 2 tsp. poppy seeds
- ¼ cup of freshly squeezed orange juice
- ½ tsp freshly grated orange rind

Directions

Combine the greens with the strawberries in a salad bowl, then set aside.

Whisk the orange juice, orange rind and poppy seeds in a separate bowl then pour over the berry-greens mixture.

Toss well to combine and serve immediately or chill in the fridge until you are ready to serve.

Enjoy!

Negative Calorie Dinner Recipes

Herbed Chicken & Veggie Stir-Fry

Yields: 4 Servings

Total Time: 20 Minutes

Preparation Time: 10 Minutes

Cook Time: 10 Minutes

Ingredients

- 4 pieces of broiled chicken breast
- 1 small bunch asparagus, ends trimmed and cut into bite size pieces
- 4 fresh garlic cloves
- 1 tbsp. Canola oil
- 1 red onion, sliced
- 1 small bunch celery, cut into bite size pieces
- 8 cherry tomatoes, cut in quarters
- 1 cup freshly chopped basil leaves
- A dash of flaxseed oil
- A dash of low-sodium soy sauce

Directions

Boil the chicken breasts until they are lightly browned and completely cooked, then set aside.

Heat the canola and flaxseed oil in a large wok and sauté the whole garlic cloves until soft condition. Add in the sliced onions, tomatoes, celery and asparagus into the garlic-flavoured oil.

Shred the boiled chicken and add it to the veggies. Add the basil leaves and stir everything together for about 3-5 minutes.

Add the soy sauce and cook for one more minute.

Serve piping hot and crisp, if you want the veggies to have a firm bite. Enjoy!

Citrusy Baked Salmon with Bulgur & Asparagus

Yields: 4 Servings

Total Time: 50 Minutes

Preparation Time: 20 Minutes

Cook Time: 30 Minutes

Ingredients

- 600g skinless salmon fillet, divided into 4 pieces
- 450g asparagus, trimmed1 ½ cups low sodium chicken or veggie broth
- 1 cup bulgur
- 2 tbsp. freshly chopped dill
- 1 lemon, thinly sliced
- ¼ tsp Kosher salt or to taste
- ¼ tsp Freshly ground black pepper to taste
- Extra virgin olive oil, for serving

Directions

Start by setting your oven to 375°F.

Combine the bulgur and broth in a shallow baking dish and season with the salt and pepper.

Gently arrange the asparagus on top in a single layer. Place the salmon fillets on top and season with salt and pepper, then top with the lemon slices.

Use foil to cover the dish tightly and bake for 30 minutes or until salmon is cooked and the asparagus and bulgur are tender.

Divide among four plates and top with chopped dill and drizzle with olive oil.

Enjoy!

Braised Chicken with Spring Veggies

Yields: 6 Servings

Total Time: 50 Minutes

Preparation Time: 20 Minutes

Cook Time: 30 Minutes

Ingredients

- 6 chicken thighs (bone-in)
- 4 carrots, cut into sticks
- 2 tbsp. freshly chopped chives
- 1 small bunch celery, cut into sticks
- 1 tbsp. olive oil
- 12 radishes, cut in half
- 1 cup low-sodium chicken broth
- Freshly ground black pepper to taste
- Kosher salt to taste

Directions

Pour the oil in a large Dutch oven over medium heat. Season the chicken with salt and pepper and add them to the Dutch oven for browning. Cook for 7 minutes or until it is evenly browned, then set aside.

Discard the excess fat from the Dutch oven and stir in the broth. Add the veggies, then top with the browned chicken and cook for about 20 minutes over medium-low heat.

Sprinkle with the chives and now you are ready to indulge yourself.

Enjoy!

The Paleo Diet Plan

What is a Paleo Approach?

A Paleo Diet, also known as the Caveman Diet, allows fruits, veggies, nuts, seeds, seafood and meat and does not allow grains, legumes, dairy, selected vegetable oils such as corn oil, soy oil and cottonseed oil. Starchy vegetables such as tubers lie in a grey area, as some Paleo followers eat them, while some people do not.

To start, the Paleo approach bans certain food that is continually marketed as 'healthy' like soy, whole grains and low-fat dairy. The main reason for this is that these foods are the major culprits behind various autoimmune diseases. This approach cleanses your body, calms your immune system, resolves all inflammation problems and helps your body to heal itself.

The Health Benefits of a Paleo Approach

The Paleo diet is one of the healthiest and most effective tools for losing weight. There are many weight loss programs, plans and diets that promise to perform wonders. What makes the Paleo approach so special?

Firstly, most of the fad weight loss diet plans, which exist nowadays, expose you to a high risk of developing some health problems and they can easily land you in a hospital bed. With these diets, you will lose weight dangerously fast, and this is a problem in and of itself. And others are just hoaxes that will only help you lose the 'water weight' and after a few weeks, all lost weight is back!

Now, let's look at the reasons that allow the Paleo Diet to be in its league:

• It doesn't ask you to take in unhealthy foods. The approach advocates for whole foods and unhealthy food does not make the cut in this diet.

• It doesn't support extreme procedures, such as intense detoxification and cleansing – the diet itself provides enough detox and cleanse.

•	Food restrictions and fasting are not part of the approach.

•	There are no counting calories or limiting the food intake.

Healthy and Sustainable Weight Loss

Every follower of the Paleo diet has experienced a massive weight loss, and the diet helps to maintain a new and healthy weight. Our ancestors used to have lean and healthy bodies. This is because the diet promotes muscle growth, better sleeping, improved metabolic processes, sufficient amount of vitamin D, good state of health, a good supply of omega-3/6 fatty acids and better stress management – all of these aspects play an important role in burning off excess body fat.

Prevention and Reduction of Chronic Disorders Symptoms

The Paleo Diet offers countless health benefits thanks to its natural and pure foods. The approach prevents arthritis, multiple sclerosis, celiac disease, heart disease, Alzheimer's disease, Crohn's disease, IBS and much more. In addition to the prevention of these diseases, the Paleo approach reduces the symptom expression of patients, who suffer from these diseases.

Detoxification

The Paleo Diet is all about consuming whole or moreover real foods with the exception of a few condiments and bottled sauces. This means that you've completely cleared hidden sugars, artificial flavourings, preservatives, colourings and hidden fats. Consequently, you fill up your system with healthy nutrients and remove all harmful toxins and chemicals from your body.

Increased nutrient intake

With the Paleo Diet, you'll remove processed carbs (which I usually refer to fillers) that actually have zero nutrition. Such food can be replaced with fresh fruits, vegetables, healthy fats, seeds and nuts, which are loaded with essential nutrients. With a healthy gut (that the diet promotes), you will have improved nutrient absorption. This is the reason why you notice that all Paleo Diet followers have strong nails, glowing skin and luscious locks – when your inside is healthy, it shows on the outside!

Clears Brain Fog

With our stressful and busy lifestyles, we experience brain fog once in a while (a condition that makes you forgetful), this is usually caused by lack of proper nourishment to your brain. You see that every part of your body, however small or big part requires to provide it with healthy meals that contain essential nutrients.

The Paleo diet is packed with essential nutrients and that's exactly what you need to jumpstart your brain!

I could go on and on with the story, how the Paleo Diet/approach is beneficial to our health, but I want you to embrace it and discover on your own the other benefits of the approach!

Three Day Paleo Diet Plan

Day 1

Breakfast: 1 Serving Ultimate Paleo Almond Flour Muffins

AM Snack: 1 apple

Lunch: 1 Serving Mustard Crusted Salmon with Arugula and Spinach Salad

PM Snack: Handful blueberries

Dinner: 1 Serving Turkey Lettuce Wraps

Day 2

Breakfast: 1 Serving Ultimate Paleo Almond Flour Muffins

AM Snack: 1 apple

Lunch: 1 Serving Mustard Crusted Salmon with Arugula and Spinach Salad

PM Snack: 1 pear

Dinner: 1 Serving Roasted Seafood w/ Herbs &Lemon

Day 3

Breakfast: 1 Serving Sausage, Leek and Asparagus, Dill Breakfast Casserole

AM Snack: Handful toasted almonds

Lunch: 1 Serving Kale, Cranberry, and Sweet Potato Salad

PM Snack: 1 glass of fresh lemon juice

Dinner: 1 Serving Grilled Lemony Chicken

Paleo Diet Breakfast Recipes

Ultimate Paleo Almond Flour Muffins

Yield: 10 Muffins

Total Time: 23 Minutes

Preparation Time: 5 Minutes

Cook Time: 18 Minutes

Ingredients

- 2-1/2 cups of almond meal or flour
- ⅓ cup of unsweetened pumpkin puree
- 3 large free-range eggs
- 2 tbsp. melted coconut oil
- 1 tsp. apple cider vinegar
- 2 tbsp. honey or maple syrup
- ½ tsp. sea salt
- ¾ tsp. baking soda
- Optional Stir-Ins: 1 cup of fresh fruit (diced apple, or blueberries)
- Optional Flavorings: citrus zest, 1 tsp. almond or vanilla extract, spice (cumin or cinnamon) or dried herbs (such as dill, basil)

Direction:

Preheat your oven to 350°F. Prepare 10 muffin cups in a standard 12-cup muffin tin by lining them with paper liners.

Whisk together almond flour, salt and baking soda (and any dried spices or herbs, if they are used).

Whisk together eggs, vinegar, extra virgin olive oil, honey and pumpkin in a small bowl (whisk in any zest or extracts at this point, if they are used).

Stir the wet ingredients into the dry mixture until it is well-blended.

Divide the batter among the prepared cups and bake for about 18 minutes or until the edges are golden brown and the centres set.

Transfer the tin to a cooling rack and let the muffins cool for at least 30 minutes before removing.

Sausage, Leek and Asparagus, Dill Breakfast Casserole

Yields: 4 to 6 Servings

Total Time: 50 Minutes

Preparation Time: 10 Minutes

Cook Time: 40 Minutes

Ingredients

- Coconut oil or butter, for greasing the dish
- 1 pound of breakfast sausage
- ¼ cup of coconut milk
- 8 free range eggs, beaten
- 1 tbsp. minced fresh dill
- 6-8 stalks asparagus, chopped
- 1 thinly sliced leek
- ¼ tsp. garlic powder
- Sea salt and pepper

Directions

Preheat your oven to 325°F. Grease a square baking dish and set aside.

Place the sausage in a pan, which is set over medium heat; break them into small pieces. Cook for a few minutes and add asparagus and leeks; continue cooking for about 5 minutes more or until sausage is no longer pink. Remove the pan from heat, discarding excess fat.

Whisk together eggs, garlic powder, dill, cream, salt and pepper in a bowl; pour the mixture into the prepared baking dish and add the sausage mixture; mix well and bake for about 40 minutes or until set in the centre.

Coconut-Blueberry Breakfast Cereal

Yields: 4 Servings

Total Time: 50 Minutes

Preparation Time: 20 Minutes

Cook Time: 30 Minutes

Ingredients

- 1/2 cup of dried blueberries
- 1/2 cup of unsweetened coconut flakes
- 1 cup of pumpkin seeds
- 2 cups of chopped pecans
- 6 medium dates, pitted
- 1/3 cup of coconut oil
- 2 tsp. cinnamon
- 1 tbsp. vanilla
- 1/2 tsp. sea salt

Directions

Preheat your oven to 325°F.

Add coconut oil, dates and half the pecans to a food processor; pulse until it is finely ground. Add pumpkin seeds and the remaining pecans and continue pulsing until it is roughly chopped.

Transfer the mixture to a large bowl and add cinnamon, vanilla and salt; spread on a baking sheet and bake for about 20 minutes or until it is browned. Remove from the oven and let cool slightly before stirring in blueberries and coconut.

Paleo Lunch Recipes

Kale, Cranberry, and Sweet Potato Salad

Yields: 6 Servings

Total Time: 20 Minutes

Preparation Time: 20 Minutes

Cook Time: 0 Minutes

Ingredients

- 2 large peeled sweet potatoes, cubed
- 2 bunches kale, chopped into small pieces
- 1 tbsp. freshly squeezed lemon juice
- 3 tbsp. extra virgin olive oil
- 1/4 cup of sunflower seeds
- 1/2 cup of dried cranberries
- 1 tsp. dijon mustard
- A pinch of sea salt
- A pinch of freshly ground pepper

Directions

Place the potatoes in a medium saucepan and cover with water; stir in a pinch of salt and bring to a gentle boil. Lower heat to a simmer and simmer for about 15 minutes or until the potatoes are tender; drain and let cool.

In a large bowl, whisk together mustard, lemon juice and extra virgin olive oil.

Add the sweet potatoes along with all the remaining ingredients; toss to mix well and serve.

Mustard Crusted Salmon with Arugula and Spinach Salad

Yields: 1 Serving

Total Time: 45 Minutes

Preparation Time: 15 Minutes

Cook Time: 20 Minutes

Ingredients

For Salmon

- 15 oz. salmon filet
- 1 tbsp. coarse ground mustard
- A pinch of sea salt

For Salad

- 2 tbsp. Dried cranberries
- 2 tbsp. chopped pecans
- 1/2 cup of chopped baby spinach
- 1 cup of chopped arugula

For Dressing

- 1 tbsp. extra virgin olive oil
- 1 tbsp. white wine vinegar

- 1 tbsp. Dijon mustard

Directions

Preheat your oven to 350°F.

Grease a baking sheet with extra virgin olive oil and place in salmon filet; pat dry with paper towels and sprinkle with ground mustard, covering the entire top of fish.

Bake for about 15 minutes or until fish flakes easily with a fork.

Meanwhile, whisk together the dressing ingredients and set aside.

Combine the salad ingredients in a mixing bowl; add in the dressing and toss until it is well-coated.

Spoon your salad onto a serving bowl and top with salmon. Enjoy!

While the salmon is cooking, whisk together the ingredients for the dressing. Set aside.

Avocado Chicken Salad

Yields: 4 Servings

Total Time: 45 Minutes

Preparation Time: 45 Minutes

Cook Time: 0 Minutes

Ingredients

- 4 boneless and skinless chicken thighs
- 3 medium avocados
- 1 tbsp. avocado oil
- 1/2 red onion, diced
- 2 small tomatoes, diced
- 1 tsp. chili powder
- 1 tsp. cumin
- Freshly squeezed lime juice from 1 lime
- A pinch of freshly ground black pepper
- A pinch of sea salt

Directions

Preheat your oven to 350°F.

Arrange chicken thighs in a baking dish and sprinkle with cumin, chilli powder and sea salt. Drizzle with extra virgin olive oil and bake for about 30 minutes or until the chicken is cooked.

Remove from oven and shred the chicken with two forks; set aside to cool.

Mash avocado in a bowl until a smooth and creamy paste is obtained. Stir in lime juice, onion and tomato until they are well-combined.

Season with salt and pepper and serve immediately.

Paleo Dinner Recipes

Turkey Lettuce Wraps

Yields: 4 Servings

Total Time: 35 Minutes

Preparation Time: 15 Minutes

Cook Time: 20 Minutes

Ingredients

- 1/2 lb. ground turkey
- 1/2 small onion, finely chopped
- 1 garlic clove, minced
- 2 tbsp. extra virgin olive oil
- 1 head lettuce
- 1 tsp. cumin
- 1/2 tbsp. fresh ginger, sliced
- 2 tbsp. freshly squeezed lime juice
- 1-2 tbsp. freshly chopped cilantro
- 1 tsp. freshly ground black pepper
- 1 tsp. sea salt

Directions

Sauté garlic and onion in extra virgin olive oil until fragrant and translucent condition.

Add turkey and cook well.

Stir in the remaining ingredients and continue cooking for 5 minutes more.

To serve, ladle a spoonful of turkey mixture onto a lettuce leaf and wrap. Enjoy!

Grilled Lemony Chicken

Yields: 2 Servings

Total Time: 6 Hours 25 Minutes

Preparation Time: 6 Hours 15 Minutes

Cook Time: 10 Minutes

Ingredients

- 1 pound of boneless and skinless chicken breasts, halved
- 1 ½ tsp. freshly minced thyme leaves
- ½ tsp. freshly ground black pepper
- ⅓ cup of extra virgin olive oil
- ⅓ cup of lemon juice, freshly squeezed
- 1 tsp. sea salt
- 2 large carrots, julienned or grated
- 1 head Romaine lettuce, bottom chiffonade leaves removed
- Nut Sauce

Directions

Whisk together extra virgin olive oil, lemon juice, thyme, sea salt and pepper in a bowl to make the marinade.

Place chicken in a baking dish; pour the marinade over the chicken and marinate in the refrigerator for at least 6 hours.

When it is ready, heat your grill and grill the chicken for about 10 minutes per side or until it is cooked.

Remove from oven, let cool and cut into small slices.

To serve, place romaine on a platter and top with carrots; place the grilled chicken over the veggies and serve with the nut sauce.

Roasted Seafood w/ Herbs &Lemon

Yields: 4 Servings

Total Time: 25 Minutes

Preparation Time: 15 Minutes

Cook Time: 10 Minutes

Ingredients

- 1/4 cup of extra virgin olive oil
- 8 scallops on the half shell
- 8 large green prawns
- 8 scampi, halved and cleaned
- 2 garlic cloves, finely chopped
- 2 tbsp. chopped flat-leaf parsley
- Finely grated lemon zest
- Freshly squeezed lemon juice from 1 lemon
- 2 tbsp. finely chopped lemon thyme

Directions

Preheat your oven to 400°F.

Arrange the seafood in a single layer in a baking dish.

Combine lemon juice, zest, garlic, extra virgin olive oil and thyme; brush over the seafood and season well.

Bake in the preheated oven for about 10 minutes or until it is cooked.

Sprinkle with chopped parsley and serve garnished with lemon wedges.

Grilled Cod with Spicy Citrus Marinade

Yields: 4 Servings

Total Time: 35 Minutes

Preparation Time: 15 Minutes

Cook Time: 20 Minutes

Ingredients

- 1 lb. cod filets
- 2 tbsp. extra virgin olive oil
- 2 minced garlic cloves
- 1/8 tsp. cayenne pepper
- 3 tbsp. freshly squeezed lime juice
- 1 ½ tsp. freshly squeezed lemon juice
- ¼ cup of freshly squeezed orange juice
- 1/3 cup of water
- 1 tbsp. finely chopped fresh thyme
- 2 tbsp. finely chopped fresh chives

Direction

In a bowl, mix lemon, lime juice, orange, cayenne pepper, extra virgin olive oil, garlic and water.

Place fish in a dish and add the marinade, reserving ¼ cup; marinate in the refrigerator for at least 30 minutes.

Broil or grill the marinated fish for about 4 minutes per side, basting regularly with the marinade.

Serve the grilled fish on a plate and top with the reserved marinade, thyme and chives.

The Whole Foods Diet

Food should nourish your entire being!

Any items of consumption that have been subjected to very minimal or preferably no processing at all refer to whole foods. The 30 Day Whole Foods Diet is based on the idea of consuming clean, fresh, healthy and natural foods to make sure of your complete and optimal physiological development.

Where it all started…

Human beings have survived on this planet for over one hundred thousand years and since the beginning of time, they have survived on natural and wild-growing foods. Our earliest ancestors thrived on wild fruits, veggies, roots and animal flesh. If Paleolithic evidence is anything to go by, they had some of the healthiest bodies.

The 30 Day Whole Foods Diet is a 30-day diet that focuses on natural foods and cuts out anything and everything processed, including even coffee. However, the only exceptions include:

•   Clarified butter and ghee

•   Vinegar

•   Fresh fruit juice

•   Snow peas, green beans and sugar snap peas because they are more 'pod' and green matter than 'grain'.

•   Salt

That's why you should embark on the 30-day whole food diet.

Increased fiber intake

The whole food diet pays greater emphasis on fruit and veggies, which are naturally endowed with fibre. Fibre plays an important role in your body by binding toxins and removing them through waste and also improving your digestive function. Some of the foods, which are rich in fibre, are almonds, broccoli, brown rice and citrus fruits.

Stay focused all day

With the whole food diet, there is no such thing as an afternoon slump, because your body is harvesting energy from high-quality sources. Natural foods provide you with a slow, but steady flow of energy that will keep you attentive and focused all day long.

Break the unhealthy chain of food addiction

"I had a terrible day, I need my favourite pick-me-up (ice cream) to cheer me up!" Does this sound like your words? With the whole food diet, you can say goodbye to your terrible food addictions and obsessions once and for all.

The whole food diet rewires your entire system and reminds every single organ in your body that it needs healthy and natural food to provide it with first-grade fuel and not empty calorie foods.

Manage and reverse symptoms of chronic illnesses

The reason, why western medicine has terribly failed at curing chronic illnesses, is that it only focuses on easing or eliminating the symptoms and not the disease or root of the issue.

A good example is, you are suffering from food sensitivity, after your appointment with your physician you are handed a box of tablets to reduce the discomfort.

The problem with this approach is that it does not address the underlying cause of inflammation, which triggered your immune system to respond with inflammation that manifested as a food sensitivity. As with any other health conditions, it starts with food!

The 30 Day Whole Food Diet is comprised of the purest and most natural foods that help your body to trigger its self-healing ability to combat even the most serious of health conditions.

Having a problem with your reproductive function?

The typical Western diet is laden with artificial ingredients that are doused with chemicals, some of which imitate the hormone estrogen. For women, the body is fooled because of thinking that there is enough estrogen and so it withholds itself from releasing estrogen therein, affecting your fertility.

Have you ever seen men with breasts or "boobs" (moobs)? This is because the estrogen-mimicking chemicals cause a higher level of 'estrogen' and as a result lower testosterone levels.

This whole food diet reboots your entire system, thus restoring normalcy in your endocrine function.

Three Day Whole Food Diet Plan

Day 1

Breakfast: 1 Serving Scotch Eggs – Chorizo Style

AM Snack: 1 banana

Lunch: 1 Serving Chinese Lettuce Wraps

PM Snack: Handful mixed berries

Dinner: 1 Serving Zoodle Sloppy Joe Bowls

Day 2

Breakfast: 1 Serving Scotch Eggs – Chorizo Style

AM Snack: 1 banana

Lunch: 1 Serving Chinese Lettuce Wraps

PM Snack: 1 apple

Dinner: 1 Serving Cauliflower Rice w/ Pork

Day 3

Breakfast: 1 Serving The green devil smoothie

AM Snack: Handful toasted walnuts

Lunch: 1 Serving Avocado and Egg salad

PM Snack: 1 glass of fresh orange juice

Dinner: 1 Serving Tasty Slow Cooker Pot Roast

The Whole Foods Diet Breakfast Recipes

Scotch Eggs – Chorizo Style

Yield: 3 Servings

Total Time: 45 Minutes

Preparation Time: 15 Minutes

Cook Time: 30 Minutes

Ingredients

- 12 ounce packages of chorizo sausage
- 12 ounce package of ground pork
- 1 jalapeno, seeded and diced
- Handful of fresh cilantro, roughly chopped
- 6 hard boiled eggs

Directions

Preheat oven to 375° degrees Fahrenheit.

Combine all of the ingredients except for the eggs in a large bowl and mix well with your hands. Divide the mixture into 6 equal pieces.

To wrap the eggs: lay a piece of plastic wrap down on your work surface. Take one portion of the pork mixture and flatten it out onto the plastic wrap. Place a hard-boiled egg in the middle and lift the plastic wrap, wrapping the egg in the sausage mixture. Repeat this action for all eggs.

Place eggs on a baking sheet and bake for 30 minutes, until sausage is cooked.

It can be served warm or cool.

Almond, Banana and Chia Pudding

Yield: 4 Servings

Total Time: 8 hours

Preparation Time: 8 hours

Cook Time: -

Ingredients

- 2 (14 ounce cans) coconut milk
- ¼ cup of chia seeds
- 2 ripe bananas, sliced
- ½ cup of toasted almonds, sliced

Directions

Open both cans of coconut milk and pour into a medium bowl. Add the chia seeds and mix thoroughly. Cover and refrigerate overnight.

By morning, the coconut/chia mixture should have thickened significantly.

Spoon into small bowls and top with sliced bananas and toasted almonds.

Serve immediately.

The Green Devil Smoothie

Yield: 1 Serving

Total Time: 10 Minutes

Preparation Time: 5 Minutes

Cook Time: 5 Minutes

Ingredients

- 1 cup of coconut milk
- ½ banana, frozen
- Handful of baby spinach
- ½ avocado
- Coconut water for desired consistency

Directions

Place the ingredients, in the listed order, in a high-speed blender.

Blend until a smooth and creamy paste is obtained. Add coconut water to thin, if it is needed.

The whole Foods Diet Lunch Recipes

Chinese Lettuce Wraps

Yield: 4 Servings

Total Time: 30 Minutes

Preparation Time: 10 Minutes

Cook Time: 20 Minutes

Ingredients

- 1 pound of ground pork
- 1 pound of mushrooms, thinly sliced
- 1 onion, chopped
- 3 cloves of garlic, minced
- 2 cups of broccoli slaw
- 2 green onions, sliced
- handful of cilantro, chopped
- 2 tablespoons of apple cider vinegar
- 2 tablespoons of fish sauce
- 2 tablespoons of coconut aminos
- 2 tablespoons of coconut oil
- Sea salt and pepper to taste
- Bibb or green leaf lettuce to serve

Directions

In a large skillet, over medium-high heat, cook the onions, garlic, and mushrooms in the coconut oil until it is tender and browned. Season with salt and pepper.

Add the ground meat and cook until it isn't pink. Stir in the apple cider vinegar, fish sauce and soy sauce.

Once the meat has cooked, lower heat to medium-low and add the broccoli slaw, green onions and cilantro. Allow the broccoli slaw to soften a bit.

To serve, scoop the mixture into lettuce cups and enjoy!

Spicy Chicken Bites

Yield: 4 Servings

Total Time: 40 Minutes

Preparation Time: 10 Minutes

Cook Time: 30 Minutes

Ingredients

- 1 pound of skinless, boneless chicken breasts
- 1 egg
- ¼ cup of water
- ¾ cup of almond meal
- 2 teaspoons of Italian seasoning
- ½ teaspoon of cayenne pepper
- ½ teaspoon of paprika
- 1 teaspoon of garlic powder
- ½ teaspoon of crushed red pepper
- ½ teaspoon of chili powder (can be adjusted to the desired level of spiciness)
- ½ teaspoon of sea salt

Directions

Preheat oven to 400° degrees. Prepare a metal baking sheet with non-stick spray.

In a medium bowl, combine the almond meal and spices. Mix well.

In a separate bowl, whisk the egg and water together.

Cut the chicken into bite-sized pieces.

Drop the chicken into the egg mixture, then transfer to the spice mixture.

Place the chicken pieces on the prepared baking sheet. Bake for 25-30 minutes, flipping halfway through until the chicken is crispy and golden-brown.

Serve immediately and store any leftovers in an airtight container in the refrigerator.

Avocado and Egg Salad

Yield: 2 Servings

Total Time: 10 Minutes

Preparation Time: 5 Minutes

Cook Time: 5 Minutes

Ingredients

- 1 ripe avocado
- 2 hard boiled eggs
- 1 small tomato
- Small bunch of cilantro (optional)
- Juice from one lemon
- Sea salt and pepper to taste

Directions

Chop the first four ingredients into small pieces.

Mix in a bowl and combine with lemon juice, salt and pepper.

Toss until it is well-combined. Serve atop salad greens, baby spinach, or even inside of

a hollowed-out tomato for a fancy
presentation.

The Whole Food Diet Dinner Recipes

Zoodle Sloppy Joe Bowls

Yield: 4 Servings

Total Time: 35 Minutes

Preparation Time: 15 Minutes

Cook Time: 20 Minutes

ingredients

- 2 tablespoons of coconut oil
- 1 red bell pepper, diced
- 1 yellow onion, diced
- 1 teaspoon of salt
- 1 teaspoon of garlic powder
- 1 pound of ground beef
- ¾ cup of homemade ketchup (recipe below)
- ¼ cup of coconut aminos
- 2 tablespoons of tomato paste
- 2 large zucchinis, spiralized

Directions

Heat the coconut oil in a large skillet over medium-high heat.

Sauté the pepper and onion in the coconut oil. Cook for about 5 minutes, until they start to soften and onions start to become translucent.

Sprinkle with salt and garlic powder and stir in.

Add the beef and break it up with a spatula. Cook until it is browned.

Add the ketchup, coconut aminos and tomato paste. Stir to combine.

Let cook on low heat for at least 10 minutes. The longer it cooks, the better flavours will develop.

Serve over zucchini noodles that have been steamed in the microwave to soften.

Cauliflower Rice w/ Pork

Yield: 4 Servings

Total Time: 50 Minutes

Preparation Time: 15 Minutes

Cook Time: 35 Minutes

Ingredients

- 2 heads of fresh cauliflower
- 1 pound of boneless skinless pork chops, diced
- 1 yellow onion, diced
- ½ green pepper, diced
- 3 tablespoons of olive oil
- 3 cloves garlic, minced
- 1 teaspoon of sea salt
- 1 teaspoon of black pepper
- ½ teaspoon of chili powder
- ½ teaspoon of dried thyme
- ¼ teaspoon of celery seed

Directions

Preheat oven to 425° degrees Fahrenheit.

Quarter the cauliflower heads and place in a food processor. Pulse several times until the cauliflower resembles rice. You may need to do this in several batches depending on the size of your food processor.

Place the riced cauliflower in a large mixing bowl. Add the pork, onion and green pepper. Toss until it is well-combined.

In a small bowl, combine the olive oil, garlic and spices. Mix well and pour over the cauliflower. Mix until everything is well coated.

Divide the rice mixture between two large baking sheets or roasting pans. Bake for 30-35 minutes, stirring halfway through. The cauliflower should be tender and browned in spots.

Tasty Slow Cooker Pot Roast

Yield: 6-8 Servings

Total Time: 5-8 hours

Preparation Time: 5-8 hours

Cook Time: 5-8 hours

Ingredients

- 2 ½ pound chuck roast or London broil
- 3 cloves of garlic, minced
- 1 yellow onion, roughly chopped
- 4-5 celery stalks, roughly chopped
- 1 cup of baby carrots
- 2 cups of homemade beef broth or water
- 3 tablespoons of fresh parsley, chopped
- Sea salt and pepper

Directions

Season your roast with salt and pepper.

Heat a large skillet over medium-high heat. Sear the roast until it is browned on all sides and add to the slow cooker.

Add the vegetables and garlic and cover with beef broth or water. (You may need to add more to ensure that it's covered.)

Cook on high heat for 5 hours or on low heat for 8 hours.

Garnish with fresh parsley and serve!

Conclusion

I would like to thank you for downloading this diet guide. I hope it has served as a great eye-opener in your approach for weight loss. You will notice that all the diets we have considered focus on fresh and natural food products.

Take your time to go through each of these diets and figure out, which one most appeals to you. If after trying one you feel as though it is not something that you can stick with, simply try another one. All of the above-listed diets have different options that are sure to appeal to a wide audience.

All the best, as you start on one of the most important journeys of your life!

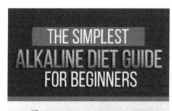
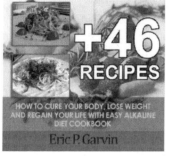

The Simplest Alkaline Diet Guide for Beginners + 46 Easy Recipes: How to Cure Your Body, Lose Weight And Regain Your Life with Easy Alkaline Diet Cookbook

Find on Amazon:
http://bit.ly/bstalkguide

Disclaimer and Terms of Use: Effort has been made to ensure that the information in this book is accurate and complete, however, the author and the publisher do not warrant the accuracy of the information, text and graphics contained within the book due to the rapidly changing nature of science, research, known and unknown facts and internet. The Author and the publisher do not hold any responsibility for errors, omissions or contrary interpretation of the subject matter herein. This book is presented solely for motivational and informational purposes.

Made in the USA
Middletown, DE
09 January 2020